Intermittent Fasting

The Uncovered Celebrity Secret To Accelerate Weight Loss, Build Lean Muscle Fast, and Secure Your Healthiest Body and Mind

James Brook

Table of Contents

Introduction

Well done and congratulations for downloading this book,

"Intermittent Fasting: The uncovered celebrity secret to accelerate weight loss, build lean muscle fast, and secure your healthiest body and mind".

This book will enlighten you on all the secrets of Intermittent Fasting, how it works, the success stories from the celebrities themselves, and how to prepare before you bring this life changing diet into your reality.

What comes to mind when you think of fat loss, young skin, a lean body and perfect health? Aren't these things in today's age one of the most sought after desires in the world, regardless of social class? Thanks to the demand, numerous solutions to a lean, youthful and healthy body have been developed. Some are way too expensive such as surgery, while others are just ridiculous, like living on strange concoctions that you can't continue using for the rest of your life.

The truth is; no one wants to keep going under the knife, even if it's to make themselves look good. Nobody wants to try the ridiculous fixes that could harm them. Everyone is looking for a natural alternative to keep the bulges away, look younger and stay healthy.

A way that balances your metabolism, induces cell repair, and does a deep cleanse of your cells, is a process called autophagy. This autophagy process is induced by a secret diet pattern called

Intermittent fasting. The American actor and former NFL player Terry Crews attests to being on this diet pattern to remain in good shape, especially since its part of his job to look good on and off screen. He says that there is no better body fix then intermittent fasting.

This book explains what intermittent fasting is and why you should actually consider it. With this book, you will realize that you don't have to become a gym junkie to look young, lean and have a perfect body. You can just modify a few aspects of your eating schedule by extending the time between meals, (unlike other diets, you don't have to change what you eat) in order to put your body in a mode where it is working towards ensuring you are lean, healthy, and have a youthful glow.

This book will help you to learn everything about intermittent fasting including what it really is, what it entails, how it works, the different celebrities who strongly advocate for it, all the health benefits, and how to do intermittent fasting in order to transform your life. Let's begin.

I want us to start on a high note to fire up your motivation to get started with intermittent fasting and make it a part of your everyday life. And what better way to do that than talk about celebrities who greatly advocate for intermittent fasting thanks to all the benefits it has brought to their lives, including having a killer magazine and beach body that many of us cannot help but drool over. Let's begin.

Intermittent Fasting: Celebrity Experience

Imagine having a job that requires you to not only stay in shape but also have to lose weight fast so that you can qualify for a role. What in the world would you do if you had to lose a certain amount of weight or get 'big enough muscles' in two months to be able to do your job? Starve yourself? Sleep in the gym working your muscles?

Well, the truth is, you would not survive long enough to play the role if you did that. Actors have to go through this all the time and they achieve it since there is no room for failure – it's their money at risk!

How do they do it? How come they don't starve or kill themselves at the gym? Well, they have a secret to their success; they found a natural and somewhat magical fix which happens when you pay attention to when you are eating.

This fix is called intermittent fasting; it is not a diet, but a diet pattern where you cycle between periods of eating and fasting. It says less about the foods you eat but emphasizes on when you eat them. There are several methods of practicing this which will be discussed in length in another chapter. Each method has a specific length of time for fasting and feeding.

Let's take a look at some celebrity testimonials about intermittent fasting

American actor and former NFL player Terry Crews and

host of Netflix's 'Ultimate Beast Master';

Terry says he has followed the diet for the last five years to stay in great shape. Needless to say, Mr. Crews is quite a muscular man. Below is a transcript from a recorded video, as he speaks about how he managed to stay in shape and feels more youthful and alive then ever before.

"Over the last five years, I've been doing intermittent fasting. What happens is, I work out very early in the morning, but then I don't eat. My first meal is at 2pm and then I eat from 2 to 10. Over the last five years, it's really kept me in great, great shape. They found, scientifically, there's a thing called "autophagy." Autophagy is when the cells in your body are rebuilding themselves. It's one of those things where you go without the food – it really strengthens your cells.

The cells are trying to rebuild, and they're trying to do their thing, and it's a wonderful thing. It's kind of like renewed. Once it's done digesting, the body's done working with food; it starts to work on other cells in the body.

I can feel the difference. I literally can put pictures of myself now versus pictures of myself at 22 years old, and I look and feel much better right now."

Other stars who have been mentioned to owe their 'smoking hot' body to this diet pattern include: Jennifer Lopez, Beyonce Knowles, Jennifer Aninston, Gwyneth Paltrow, Victoria Secret's angel Miranda Kerr and late night TV host Jimmy Kimmel. They have sung praises about how intermittent fasting has helped them to keep themselves looking the way they do - hot. Another actor named Benedict Cumberbatch has been using the same eating pattern to stay in shape for his role as Sherlock Holmes in the Sherlock Holmes sequel. He confessed in an interview with

Caitlin Moran for the times, 'I'm on the 5:2 diet...' (5:2 is code for a certain type of intermittent fasting)

Several Cast members of the Coronation Street have tried out the diet. Ian Puleston who plays Owen Armstrong has lost a stone on the diet pattern, which is said to have inspired other members such as Cherylee Houston who plays Izzy Armstrong, to try it out. Phillip Schofield the 'This Morning' star, lost 9lbs in four weeks thanks to intermittent fasting.

If this diet pattern is good enough for a model such as Miranda Kerr, and Jennifer Lopez whose body and looks are age defying (you cannot believe she is in her late forties), and the slaying queen Beyonce (who has got the body plus the moves to die for), it must be good.

What does this diet do for them so well, that they can confidently swear by it? What does it do to their body and how is it this beneficial?

Find out in the next chapter.

The Benefits Of Intermittent Fasting And The Science Behind Its Success

How will you benefit from adopting a fasting and feeding routine? To explain this, we shall discuss the various changes and happenings that occur within the bodies of those who fast, and how these changes are not only beneficial for your appearance, but more importantly for your overall health and well-being.

What Happens When You Fast?

Many of us believe that fasting or rather not eating puts the body in starvation mode, lowers your energy levels, and could cause your body system to crash. This is why if you tell someone you are on a diet that calls for you to go without food for some 16 hours or more, most people will think you're crazy or your trying to starve yourself. They will tell you that you have chosen a hopeless path. How right could they be? What actually goes on in the body when you don't eat?

The first point to note is that the changes that happen in the body when you fast, entirely depend upon the length of the continuous fast.

After about 12-14 hours of fasting, the body enters into the 'fasted state'. The body uses the 12-14 hours to digest and absorb nutrients from the gut, and then uses this nutrients inside of the bloodstream. By around this time, all the nutrients that were absorbed into the bloodstream have been used up, and the body has already started using up glycogen (a stored form of glucose, which acts as a temporary source of energy for times like these i.e.

when you have not had food for an extended period). The glycogen is created from glucose during the 'fed state', but if you don't eat for a considerably long period (roughly 12-14hours), the body will start automatically using this glycogen storage for energy.

To help you understand this, let's take a step back and talk about all the events that happen when you eat food.

When you eat, the body spends the next few hours (3-5 hours) digesting the food that you just ate. This is the time it breaks down different macronutrients into different absorbable molecules. For instance, glucose is produced when carbohydrates are broken down, fatty acids are the product of the breakdown of fats, where as amino acids are the product of the breakdown of proteins in the digestive system. It takes another 5-8 hours to actually absorb what you've broken down and use it up for various bodily processes.

When all the food is gone and your stomach is empty, a hormone called ghrelin is released. The main function of this hormone is to prepare the body to find something to eat. It is also responsible for causing other hormones that stimulate lipolysis (fat release from adipose cells) to be released. The more ghrelin is produced, the hungrier you get – your body is being urged to find food/a source of energy. Epinephrine, the hormone responsible for your metabolism is also released at this point and your resting metabolism rises as your body screams, 'You need to eat!' Many of us heed to the body's call for us to eat because we are hungry. But remember that during this time, the body still has a lot of energy in the bloodstream, which it is yet to use.

It takes about 12-14 hours from the last meal before the body can actually be in real need for food. Eating earlier than this will only make the body stay in a fed state all the time, which is not healthy, as this state is characterized by fat storage. How is that so? Well, when glucose (the product of the breakdown of carbohydrates) gets into the bloodstream, the body releases insulin from the pancreas to help the cells take up the glucose for use or storage. The role of insulin in this case is to act as some sort of key that opens up the doors to the cells.

This happens in order to make the cells actually able take up glucose, because the cells don't actually have their own internal mechanism for absorbing glucose from their environment. In fact, without insulin, the cells could die of high levels of blood sugar (it increases acidity in the bloodstream) and starve to death because they cannot absorb glucose - this is like a case of diabetes where blood sugar levels shoot up too high because of inefficiencies in the production or use of insulin. Since our normal diet tends to be high in carbohydrates (assuming we follow the USDA recommended food pyramid), this essentially means that we are likely to have more glucose than what the cells need in the bloodstream.

Since the role of insulin is to keep directing glucose into the cells, if its concentration is still high, the cells start storing this excess by having it transported to the liver for conversion to glycogen, which is then stored in the liver and muscle cells. This glycogen acts like a backup source of power that is always readily available if the need arises, e.g. when you engage in strenuous physical activities or when you go on an extended fast.

Glycogen stores are limited though; they can take just about 2000kcal of energy at any particular time so when these are filled, the excess needs an alternative (preferably an unlimited) storage space. The different fat stores around the body provide this unlimited storage space. For the glucose to qualify for storage, it is first converted into fatty acids and glycerol, before being moved on to the fat stores. The more you deposit into the fat stores, the more weight you gain. All these things can take place during the 'fed state'.

The 'fasted state' reverses the body's energy storage mechanisms. For starters, when dietary glucose is depleted, the body secretes another hormone, glucagon from the pancreas. The role of this hormone is to trigger the liver to convert glycogen into glucose for use as energy. The body doesn't metabolize all the glycogen though; given that some processes within the body can only run on glucose, it spares some of the glycogen for use in fueling key body processes that only run on glucose. Since there is a resultant drop in insulin levels, the fat cells start releasing the fatty acids and glycerol, which are then metabolized in the liver in a series of processes that supply the body with energy.

As much as 60-70 percent of the body's cells can run on energy from your fat metabolism when you are in the 'fasted state'. The remaining 30-40 percent runs on glucose, which can be supplied from the glycogen stores and from the breakdown of other non carb sources, such as proteins and glycerol. The body however, doesn't start using up proteins until after an extended fast of about 72 hours of being in the 'fasted state'. Intermittent fasting doesn't get you past the 36 hour mark so you have no reason to worry!

With a prolonged fast of many days and weeks, if you eventually hit the three weeks mark your body will go into 'starvation mode', which is basically your body breaking down most of its protein and muscle for energy. When the muscles are gone, the body only has tissues to convert to energy. This is the danger zone of fasting as before the tissues are broken down, the lack of essential nutrients and vitamins already compromises your immunity. You may become ill or fall into a vegetative state followed by death. No one should ever get to this point- at least not willingly as they will probably not live to tell the story (pun intended).

The intermittent fasting protocols that we shall discuss soon will never get your body into starvation mode, given that it allows you to break your fasts. The longest fasted period is 36 hours. It gives you a gentle transition from using glucose for energy, to breaking down fat, without going to the extremes where muscle is broken for protein. It will only get you to the point where you burn fat, have less cholesterol, and your cells are renewing through the process of autophagy.

All these processes that take place during the 'fasted state' bring about rapid weight loss, as well as many other benefits, which we will discuss next.

What Benefits Does The Body Get From The Above? (The Healthy Part)

It gets a chance to cleanse and renew cells through autophagy to prevent aging.

Autophagy comes from two Greek words namely 'auto', which literally means 'self', and 'phagy' which when translated means 'eating'; therefore, the word autophagy in simple terms can be taken to mean self-eating. It is a normal physiological process in the body that deals with recycling, renewing and destruction of cells.

Through this, the body manages to clean out debris which include toxins. It maintains normal functioning of the body at a cellular level, by protein degradation and recycling of the destroyed cell organelles to make new cells.

The process of autophagy kicks in and operates at maximum during cellular stress. Among the causes of cellular stress is deprivation of nutrients or growth factors. This can be done through fasting – fasting is a biological stressor.

How will you benefit from this?

Autophagy is the ultimate anti-aging fix. During cellular cleansing, the body identifies old and substandard cellular parts and marks them for destruction – it clears out all of the old junk accumulated in the cells. This is what gives you that youthful abundance of life. No wonder Jennifer Lopez looks so young!

The accumulation of this junk is the reason why you look aged! The autophagy process when you're fasting gives your body a complete renovation make over! It's like you buy an old home, but then replace the old junk with new furniture and paint, and make it look brand new!

Protection From Diseases- Lifestyle Diseases

Even the high and mighty, and the rich and famous, can develop diseases from a poor choice of lifestyle. How many celebrities have been reported to have died suddenly from a heart attack or to be long suffering with cancer, blood pressure and diabetes?

They have discovered that there is better prevention and possible cure for all those ailments, a cure that no doctor can give and they don't have to pay for it. - Intermittent fasting. With this fix, they can not only look younger, but also stay healthy, so they can continue doing whatever they want to do. Whether it's singing and dancing, acting or sports, pulling off those movie stunts, all of these things require them to have a healthy body. - As everything in life does.

Does fasting really help in preventing or curing lifestyle diseases? Let's find out.

To explain this, I will start by quoting the Greek physician Hippocrates:

"Everyone has a physician inside him or her; we just have to help

it in its work. The natural healing force within each one of us is the greatest force in getting well. Our food should be our medicine. Our medicine should be our food. But to eat when you are sick is to feed your sickness."

For thousands of years, even during those days when obese people were rare (there were no Burger Kings and fried chicken on every corner), therapeutic fasting was a common healing protocol for many diseases. Famous people such as Aristotle and the aforementioned Hippocrates knew the value of missing a meal especially when ill.

It is strange that 'not eating' is a natural response for most people and animals when they fall ill. Cancer patients undergoing chemotherapy find it hard to eat – we take it as a nasty side effect of cancer. Even animals like cats and dogs that usually have voracious appetites, will stop eating for a while upon falling ill. I am of the opinion that there is a physiological explanation why the body behaves this way.

We think this lack of appetite is bad, or is proof that we are actually getting worse. We do anything to force food down our throats, apparently to survive. Could it be that the body switches on the 'lack of appetite' mode to activate our inner physician? Would it be of help if we just didn't eat for a while? Maybe so.

Let me explain how fasting helps prevent and cure some of the common maladies.

- **Alzheimer's Disease And Dementia**

The accumulation of dirt, such as the old junk proteins in cells, can result into Alzheimer's disease and dementia. Actually, the greatest risk factor of this disease is aging. It is a disease of the brain caused by the accumulation of abnormal protein over the years, which gums up the brain system. When this protein is cleared and new brain cells are regenerated through the process of autophagy, the development of this disease could be inhibited.

Also, as discussed earlier, intermittent fasting helps slow aging. If it could do this, it is possible that it can delay age related diseases such as this.

- **Cancer**

Fasting fights cancer in different ways:

-Starves cancer cells

According to a cancer researcher from USC Valter Longo, when normal cells are starved of energy and nutrients, they go into survival mode. They behave like an animal in hibernation mode; they will lay low and display extreme resistance to stressors until they are able to feed normally again. Cancer cells are not able to do that. They stay 'on' functioning at their maximum with a 'goal' to grow, reproduce and consume resources, which they do not realize are no longer there. Eventually, they can no longer feed since they can only convert glucose for energy (which gets depleted) and not other sources like ketone bodies or fat, like normal cells.

-Puts normal cells into 'survival mode'

Longo studied increased cellular resistance in response to oxidative stress, a phenomenon that arises during fasting. He figured that chemotherapy induced oxidative stress to both cancerous and normal cells. Fasting caused normal cells to go into survival mode. With further research on mice, he found that by going into survival mode, normal cells would be protected from the effects of chemotherapy. This leaves the fully operational cancer cells exposed to the treatment, if the patient has fasted.

"...Tumor-ridden mice were either fasted or fed normally 48 hours prior to a large does of chemotherapy. Half of the

normally-fed mice died from chemotherapy toxicity, while all of the fasted mice survived. Furthermore, fasting did not improve the survival rate of cancerous cells, meaning it only protected normal, healthy cells." -Valter Longo's study.

He concluded that fasting is likely to improve the condition of cancer patients by lessening the side effects of chemotherapy, and exposing only the cancer cells to the treatment and sparing the normal ones.

-Improves insulin sensitivity

Intermittent fasting regulates the levels of blood sugar therefore improving insulin sensitivity and reducing insulin resistance, which have been directly linked to several cancers such as breast, prostate and pancreatic.

Diabetes, Obesity And Cardiovascular Disease

-Aids in weight loss

Obesity, diabetes and cardiovascular disease are intimately linked, especially abdominal obesity. Losing this weight could be of great help for a patient suffering from any of these conditions. However, the dilemma is how to lose weight, since if you are already suffering from these conditions, there are methods that will be risky for you.

According to Canadian nephrologists Dr. Jason Fung, intermittent fasting coupled with a low carb high fat diet, is an effective method for weight loss for people with or without diabetes or cardiovascular diseases. Lessening the amount of calories and giving your body time to deplete glycerol stores and start burning fat, is the simplest and fastest way of losing fat – fasting forces the body to burn fat when the normal glucose from ingested food is not available. Note that, it's not just any kind of fasting as this could be dangerous – it should be controlled fasting with feeding and fasting periods such as intermittent fasting.

-Helps lower bad cholesterol

High level of bad cholesterol is a risk factor for cardiovascular disease such as heart attacks and stroke. Note that cholesterol is not a form of stored fat that can be burned for energy. It is a substance used for cellular repair in cell walls and also makes certain hormones. 80% of the cholesterol in our blood is produced by the liver, thus reducing the amount of dietary cholesterol has no effect on the levels in the blood.

Fasting could be the key to lowering blood cholesterol. Bad cholesterol (LDL) can be lowered by controlled 'starvation' such as intermittent fasting.

Hormone Control

Most bodily functions are made possible by hormones. You could control and regulate hormones to use them to your advantage.

-Insulin

Controlled fasting helps manage insulin. This is the hormone that regulates blood sugar. High levels of insulin over an extended period can make cells develop resistance to the hormone. Think of having to hear loud noises all the time; you get to a point where your hearing is impaired, right? That's what happens when you constantly bombard your body with high carb foods that are normal in our everyday life, coupled with our 'eat six small meals' mantra, which keeps our insulin levels high all the time. It also promotes fat storage in fat cells and therefore it is possible that with such high levels, you will gain weight. When we eat, insulin levels rise and they drop when we fast (I mean when we get to the fasted state), as there is not so much glucose in the blood. Insulin resistance in cells is the major cause of diabetes type 2 and obesity.

Adopting intermittent fasting as a lifestyle, for instance having a 16 hour fasting period daily, helps keep this hormone in check; at low/normal levels thus normalizing cells sensitivity to it. This is important for optimal health since insulin resistance is a primary contributing factor to chronic diseases such as cancer, diabetes and cardiovascular disease.

-Human Growth Hormone (HGH)

Fasting triggers a rise in the human growth hormone. The HGH is commonly referred to as the 'fitness hormone'. This hormone plays a major role in maintaining health and fitness, by promoting muscle growth and boosting fat loss by increasing your metabolism. It is the hormone that tells your body to burn fat for energy when the glycogen stores get depleted. It helps you lose weight/fat without sacrificing muscle mass. This is the key to becoming lean, not thin – you retain muscle but lose fat. This must be the secret for athletes who despite having gigantic muscles, are still fit and swift.

Ghrelin hormone

Otherwise referred to as the hunger hormone, ghrelin is secreted in the stomach when it starts getting empty. The hungrier you are, the higher its levels in the blood. Ghrelin is the main driving force behind the enhanced secretion of the Human Growth Hormone discussed above. Also, it has been said to improve cognitive abilities as it seems to promote the growth of brand new brain cells as well as protect them from the effects of aging. What better way to ensure an increased production of the hunger hormone and subsequent production of HGH, than to fast for an extended period?

Fasting promotes longevity

Longevity means long life. Who wants to die young anyway? I am sure everybody wants to live and enjoy a long life. It is said that we eat to live – to live long I suppose. However, could it be that we are digging early graves by 'eating to live' all the time, and eating less often is the secret to living longer?

Fasting has been found to lengthen the lifespan of lab mammals and improve health markers associated with aging and longevity, in both animals and humans. There hasn't been proof yet on how it increases longevity in humans, since no studies have been conducted on humans. However, by reducing the risk of major killer diseases such as diabetes, hypertension, heart attack and cancer, it has somewhat reduced your risk of dying; the fewer things you have trying to kill you, the longer you are likely to live!

It is clear that intermittent fasting is the way to go. But before you do, let's learn a few things about the diet so that you know exactly what you're getting yourself into.

Everything You Need To Know About Intermittent Fasting Before You Try It.

If you have read this far, you know that this is a diet pattern you ought to make a lifestyle out of. If you do this you'll never have to worry about fat bulges in the wrong places again. You'll bring a new refreshed level of health and youthfulness into your life through this anti-aging process. You may even prevent or cure some of the chronic lifestyle diseases that plague today's society. However, before you make a commitment to start fasting this way, there are a few facts about this diet that you need to know so that you can do this right, be safe, and reap the most benefits.

Note: The things we shall discuss here are answers to some frequently asked questions about this diet. Read on and be in the know:

What really is Intermittent fasting?

As mentioned before, Intermittent fasting is a diet/eating pattern where you cycle between periods of eating and fasting. The length of the fasting period depends on your choice model of IF but ideally, you should be aiming to do at least 14 hours without taking any calorie rich foods or drinks, if you want to get into the 'fasted state'. You can extend your fast to as long as 36 hours if you desire, depending on what your goals are. We will discuss the different intermittent fasting protocols later on in the book.

A point to note about this pattern is that it does not emphasize on the supposed importance of breakfast everyone talks about. Actually, it is easier for you to follow through if you make breakfast time to be part of your fasting time. Many people do not agree. However, the following explanation may make you agree with me:

Most of us freak out and count ourselves out when we hear the word 'fasting'. Our 'eat three meals a day' tradition causes many to look at fasting as an alien and harmful practice. However, the truth is that fasting is not alien or hard. Actually, you would be surprised if I told you that you practice it as often as every single day! When you are not eating, you are fasting; when you sleep, you do not eat; therefore, you are fasting! Isn't it easier to fast when you are sleeping, when you are unconscious of the fact that you are missing out on food? The thing is; many of us cannot ignore food when we can see it, which is what makes it hard to recommend that someone avoids food, when they can see the food. Sleep fasting is much easier. You are only required to make a small extension into your awake/conscious hours; you simply push the time you 'break-fast' (breakfast simply means breaking your sleeping fast). This is why for intermittent fasting, missing breakfast is quite beneficial.

Who is/is not eligible to practice intermittent fasting?

Is this diet pattern for everyone? Unfortunately, although intermittent fasting is good for your health and general well being, not everyone can fast. There are groups of people whom it would harm. They are:

- People suffering from type 1 diabetes, anorexia nervosa, or bulimia nervosa cannot do any form of IF(intermittent fasting).

- Those suffering from type 2 diabetes can practice it, but only under medical supervision because they are on insulin medication which may need some adjustment.

Remember IF affects insulin levels in the blood and so does the medication thus the need for medical advice.

- Pregnant women, breast feeding mothers, and children in their bloom years should avoid intermittent fasting. These groups of people require lots of energy and thus they cannot afford to be deprived of any nutrients at any point.

- People suffering from eating disorders, adrenal disorders, depression and insomnia, ought to be treated for their conditions before they try to fast.

If you find yourself eligible to practice intermittent fasting, use the following tips when you get started. They will help you cope and attain your goals.

- *Do not plan or imitate; listen to your body*

When it comes to choosing an IF diet plan to follow, do not imitate a friend or plan for one, may be because it sounds good or comfortable – do not make any assumptions on what can or cannot work for you. Listen to your body.

Intermittent fasting works best when it is done naturally; if you force yourself, you may end up overeating or binging after the fast. Also, do not compare yourself with anyone; what worked for someone else may not work for you – bodies and metabolism are different.

If skipping breakfast seems too crazy for you, then have breakfast and plan your fasting hours with that in consideration. For instance, if you are on a 16hour fast, you can have your feeding period from 8.00am to 4.00 pm and fast till 8.00 am the next day. This means that you will eat breakfast and not struggle through your day in the name of fasting.

- *Start slow*

It is impossible to come from having six meals a day to having one meal. As mentioned above, this pattern should come naturally. Do not restrict or deprive yourself. Take it slow; you can start by avoiding snacking in between meals then move on skipping regular meals. Wean yourself off having six meals a day, by having four, then to three, as you cut them down to what fits your diet pattern. Your body will get adapted to having lesser glucose, then it will also adapt itself to burning fat. You will notice that once you get fat-adapted, you will feel less hungry. Then you will be able to get through your fasting period without awful hunger pains.

- *Keep yourself busy*

It will not be easy to skip meals when you spend all day next to the kitchen or on the sofa right opposite the fridge where you kept tasty cupcakes. Even if you do not feel hungry, you will get tempted to treat yourself to some snacks if you are surrounded by food. A busy schedule is likely to keep you away from food temptations.

- *Stay away from white coffee/bullet proof coffee/ butter coffee*

Some types of IF allow you to take coffee or tea during the fasting period. Many people think that just taking any coffee and tea with 'healthy creams' is okay. Note that ingesting butter or coconut oil, or adding any other cream or sweetener to your tea or coffee, will not maintain your fasted state. Anything with any caloric value will have the same effect as food. If you have to take coffee or tea, keep it black like the ultimate keto coffee.

- *Do not expect that fasting will fix everything*

Knowing the benefits of intermittent fasting, it is likely you have very high expectations of what it can deliver you. It can potentially help you to lose weight and fight disease, but you should also know that it is just but one of several factors that can help you to achieve your goal. Other important factors include exercise, good nutrition (eat healthy foods during feeding period), and good quality sleep that rejuvenates the body, mind and spirit.

You should not use this diet pattern as a quick fix when you eat excess carbs all the time, or as a substitution for exercise.

- *Drink enough water*

There is no good nutrition without water, given that a great percentage of our bodies comprises of water. Make sure that you take enough water to keep yourself hydrated, even during your fasting period for a healthier outcome. Also, water will be able to 'drown' the hunger pains, as sometimes our body communicates 'thirst' and we understand 'hunger'.

With all we've learnt so far, I believe that you are now ready to try Intermittent fasting. So how exactly do you go about it? That's what we will discuss next.

How To Do Intermittent Fasting; A Step By Step Guide

There is no one method that is perfect for everyone. People have varying metabolisms, schedules and preferences. Also in the previews chapter, we have mentioned that it is advisable to practice this naturally, by doing what your body is comfortable with. Everyone could have their own way of practicing IF, but it is important to have guiding principles that are provided by the various protocols of IF - the several ways of practicing intermittent fasting. Note that, you can choose the one that works best for you and adjust it to fit your schedule, so long as the fasting and feeding windows remain constant. Let me guide you through them.

The Lean gains Protocol

This is an IF method that is characterized by a 14hour or 16 hour fast, followed by an 8 hour or 10 hour feeding window. For example, if you have your last meal (dinner) at 8.00pm, you fast through the night and extend into the morning, where you push your breakfast/lunch (whichever name you want to call your first meal) to a few hours after you wake up; at 12.00 noon if your fasting period is 16hours and 10.00am if its 14 hours.

During the fasted period, the lean gains protocol does not allow you to consume any calories. However, in the beginning, you can have black coffee with sugar-free sweeteners, diet soda or sugar-free gum.

Note that, you are required to maintain a constant feeding time; try to feed at the same time everyday to avoid throwing your hormones (which respond to the presence of food) out of whack/into confusion, which can interfere with several body processes such as menstruation for women. During the feeding window, ensure that you eat whole unprocessed foods or a protein shake/meal replacement bar when you do not have time for food.

Tips to cope

Lean gains requires you to exercise, preferably just before breaking your fast. Your meal plan depends on your workout schedule. On the days you exercise you ought to eat more carbs than fat, while on rest days fat is more important. On either days; rest or workout, your protein consumption should be fairly high (the quantities are determined by factors such as gender, age, body fat and activity levels).

The Warrior Diet

This diet pattern requires you to adopt a warrior like lifestyle. Traditional warriors spent their day either in battle, or doing patrols to keep away enemies from their communities – this means they were engaged in rigorous activity all day. These warriors, due to their nature of work, needed to be alert at all times, and they did not have three or six meals a day – protecting a community does not give you such a luxury. They only ate one large meal in the evening and maybe raw fruits or vegetables in the wilderness. The warrior diet is created around this kind of lifestyle. It requires you to fast for 20 hours and have a four hour feeding window in the evening.

During the 20 hour fast, you are allowed to eat a few servings of low carb raw vegetables and fruits, fresh juice or protein if desired. This usually maximizes your body's fight or flight response of the sympathetic nervous system to stimulate fat burning, boost energy and promote alertness.

During the feeding window, you have to be mindful of what you eat and the order in which you eat it. This is meant to make digestion easier for the body since you are eating everything at once. Start off with the vegetables/fruits, carbohydrates (very few), then move on to proteins, and then finish with fat.

FAQ answered

Many people ask, why eat at night when the body does not require much energy; wouldn't this mean that you are storing more fat? Let me explain.

When you eat at night, you activate the parasympathetic nervous system, which helps put the body into relaxation mode. It promotes calmness, relaxation, and digestion, while allowing the body to use nutrients for repair and growth. Also, feeding at night may help the body produce hormones that help burn fat during the day, according to the founder Hofmekler.

Eat Stop Eat (24 Hour Fast)

This diet pattern is commonly referred to as the 5:2 fast diet. You are supposed to eat normally for 5 days and fast two inconsecutive days. You cannot consume any food during the 24 hour fast but calorie-free beverages are allowed.

When the fast is over, you can go back to normal eating – 'normal' is emphasized because most people go back to overeating to compensate for fasting, and end up eating so many calories. The founder of Eat Stop Eat, Pilon says to 'act like you didn't fast'. This diet is intended to create a calorie deficit without limiting what you eat but when you eat it. For efficiency a regular workout, particularly resistance training, is a major component of the 5:2

fast.

Tips to cope

Since the fasting days are not fixed, this gives you the flexibility to choose your fast days. It is advisable to schedule these days for when you are busy. It is not easy to go for 24 hours without food on a weekend while relaxing in the house or attending parties. Also, to make coping through the fasts easier, stay hydrated by taking lots of water - you will feel less hungry.

Up Day Down Day (Alternate Day Fasting)

This intermittent fasting method requires you to eat very little one day and eat normally the next day. On the down days, you eat very little, which means you reduce your daily calorie intake to only 500 calories. On the up days, you eat normally, which means you consume your normal daily calorie requirement for instance 2000 calories.

It is easy to over consume calories on down days (especially when you are starting out) thus the founder, James Johnson recommends that you go for meal replacement shakes, which you can sip throughout the day instead of having many small meals. However, you can only do this during the first two weeks as you adapt to the diet, but you should start consuming real foods soon after.

If you have a workout schedule (which you should), you may find it harder to hit the gym on the low calorie days; you may run out of energy fast. It would be smart if you could have it easy on these days and save the hard work out days for the up days.

Tips to cope

Plan your meals ahead of time to avoid overeating/binging on your normal feeding days, when your belly is grumbling after a day of under eating. Plan ahead because the day when you can eat, you will want to eat everything.

But just remember, success tastes sweeter then anything.

Conclusion

And with that we have come to the end of the book. Thank you and congratulations for reading until the end, I hope you enjoyed it.

Now you should have a much deeper understanding of what intermittent fasting is, how it works, and what a difference it can make in your life. The next step is to apply what you've learned from this and put it into your daily routine. The best way to see the results for yourself is always to take action. Watch what an amazing transformation it will make to your health, your weight, and not to mention that glowing youthful vitality, inside and out.

Finally, if you enjoyed this book, it would be greatly appreciated if you could share your thoughts and leave an Amazon review for me!

Thank you and good luck!